Cristian Andrei Sarau
Marioara Poenaru
Nicolae Constantin Balica

Wegener's Granulomatosis in ENT Department Timisoara

Cristian Andrei Sarau
Marioara Poenaru
Nicolae Constantin Balica

Wegener's Granulomatosis in ENT Department Timisoara

LAP LAMBERT Academic Publishing

Impressum / Imprint

Bibliografische Information der Deutschen Nationalbibliothek: Die Deutsche Nationalbibliothek verzeichnet diese Publikation in der Deutschen Nationalbibliografie; detaillierte bibliografische Daten sind im Internet über http://dnb.d-nb.de abrufbar.

Alle in diesem Buch genannten Marken und Produktnamen unterliegen warenzeichen-, marken- oder patentrechtlichem Schutz bzw. sind Warenzeichen oder eingetragene Warenzeichen der jeweiligen Inhaber. Die Wiedergabe von Marken, Produktnamen, Gebrauchsnamen, Handelsnamen, Warenbezeichnungen u.s.w. in diesem Werk berechtigt auch ohne besondere Kennzeichnung nicht zu der Annahme, dass solche Namen im Sinne der Warenzeichen- und Markenschutzgesetzgebung als frei zu betrachten wären und daher von jedermann benutzt werden dürften.

Bibliographic information published by the Deutsche Nationalbibliothek: The Deutsche Nationalbibliothek lists this publication in the Deutsche Nationalbibliografie; detailed bibliographic data are available in the Internet at http://dnb.d-nb.de.

Any brand names and product names mentioned in this book are subject to trademark, brand or patent protection and are trademarks or registered trademarks of their respective holders. The use of brand names, product names, common names, trade names, product descriptions etc. even without a particular marking in this work is in no way to be construed to mean that such names may be regarded as unrestricted in respect of trademark and brand protection legislation and could thus be used by anyone.

Coverbild / Cover image: www.ingimage.com

Verlag / Publisher:
LAP LAMBERT Academic Publishing
ist ein Imprint der / is a trademark of
OmniScriptum GmbH & Co. KG
Heinrich-Böcking-Str. 6-8, 66121 Saarbrücken, Deutschland / Germany
Email: info@lap-publishing.com

Herstellung: siehe letzte Seite /
Printed at: see last page
ISBN: 978-3-659-78242-8

Copyright © 2015 OmniScriptum GmbH & Co. KG
Alle Rechte vorbehalten. / All rights reserved. Saarbrücken 2015

WEGENER GRANULOMATOSIS IN ENT DEPARTMENT TIMISOARA

CRISTIAN ANDREI SARĂU[1],
MARIOARA POENARU[2]
NICOLAE CONSTANTIN BALICA[2]

[1]DEPARTMENT OF MEDICAL SEMIOLOGY I, "VICTOR BABEȘ" UNIVERSITY OF MEDICINE AND PHARMACY, TIMISOARA, ROMANIA

[2]DEPARTMENT OF ENT, "VICTOR BABEȘ" UNIVERSITY OF MEDICINE AND PHARMACY, TIMISOARA, ROMANIA

WEGENER GRANULOMATOSIS IN ENT DEPARTMENT TIMISOARA

TABLE OF CONTENT

WEGENER GRANULOMATOSIS IN ENT DEPARTMENT TIMISOARA	page 7
WEGENER'S GRANULOMATOSIS	page 8
Epidemiology/aetiology	page 9
Symptoms	page 9
Diagnosis	page 19
Differential diagnosis	page 36
Pathology	page 38
Treatment	page 42
Prognosis	page 48
CONCLUSION	page 49
REFERENCES	page 50

WEGENER GRANULOMATOSIS IN ENT DEPARTMENT TIMISOARA

The authors present their experience regarding Wegener's granulomatosis in patients addressed to the ENT Department Timisoara, "Victor Babes" University of Medicine and Pharmacy Timisoara, Romania.

The patients presented a multiorganic manifestation aspect of Wegener's granulomatosis. The main symptoms were in ENT field, involving upper-airway.

The diagnosis of Wegener's granulomatosis was established on the suspicion of Ear Nose and Throat (ENT) clinical exam. The exams that followed, represented by other tests and investigations were performed in the ENT Department and Department of Medical Semiology I (nephrology, internal medicine and dermatology).

All the patients presented multiorganic involvement.

As a particular aspect we noted the prolonged evolution in a stable condition in one patient out of the 4 cases.

WEGENER'S GRANULOMATOSIS

In 1939 Friedrich Wegener defined for the first time Wegener's granulomatosis as a systemic disease. Wegener's granulomatosis is characterized by necrotizing granulomas with systemic vasculitis, mainly involving the upper and lower respiratory tract and renal involvement represented by focal necrotizing or proliferative glomerulonephritis (Wegener F, 1939).

Wegener's granulomatosis, being a rare multisystem autoimmune disease, has an unknown aetiology (Rossini BAA, et. al., 2010)(Scalcon MRR, et. al. 2008).

It is a systemic vasculitis, affecting small and medium-sized vessels of the upper and lower respiratory tract and kidneys, including necrotizing granulomas (Scalcon MRR, et. al. 2008) (Antunes T, Barbas CSV., 2005).

Wegener's granulomatosis is clinically represented by recurrent respiratory infection, renal manifestations, and nonspecific systemic symptoms.

The classic triad of Wegener's granulomatosis organ involvement is represented by: the upper respiratory tract, lower respiratory tract (lungs) and kidneys.

In most cases the first location of manifestation is the nose, but it can also occur in the middle ear, the oral cavity, larynx and the oropharynx. (Bailey B., 2006)(Cummings C., 2005).

In ENT Wegener's granulomatosis is not a common disease.

After 2012, with the advent of a new Chapel Hill Consensus Conference (CHCC 2012), it was renamed granulomatosis with polyangiitis (Jennette JC, et. al., 2013).

Since 2013, due to the recommendations of the American College of Rheumatology (ACR), the American Society of Nephrology (ASN) and the European League Against Rheumatism (EULAR), a new Chapel Hill Consensus Conference (CCHC2012) updated the classification of Wegener's granulomatosis to granulomatosis with polyangiitis, in order to optimize the official system of classification of vasculitis and to identify a more suitable criteria for classification and diagnosis (Jennette JC, et. al., 2013).

Epidemiology/aetiology

Wegener's granulomatosis is a rare disease.

It affects about 1 in 20,000–30,000 people (3 cases per 100,000, and the mean age at diagnosis is 55 years (Cotch MF et al., 1996)). The highest prevalence is in middle-aged Caucasian patients, but any age might be interested. Men and women are similarly affected, nor is there any evidence for a hereditary element. More than 90% of all patients with Wegener's granulomatosis are white. The remaining 1% to 4% of patients are African-American, Hispanic, or Asian (Seo P, Stone JH, 2004).

With an unknown etiology, has no gender preferences, common in Caucasians, with undetermined worldwide incidence (Taborda P, Taborda V., 1998) (Brandt HR, et. al., 2009).

In the United States it is estimated 3 cases per 100,000 people, and in the United Kingdom, 109 cases per million inhabitants (Chung L, et. al., 2008) (Taborda P, Taborda V., 1998).

Symptoms

The disease may present with

- pulmonary
- upper respiratory tract
- renal involvement

At initial presentation 45% of patients have a pulmonary affection, while during the late phase's raises to 87% of patients. (Fauci AS, et. al., 1983) (Cordier JF, et. al., 1990).

Wegener's granulomatosis initial signs and symptoms first interest the ENT area, followed by lung, skin, and kidneys (Antunes T, Barbas CSV., 2005) (Correa JC, et. al., 1985).

Wegener's granulomatosis may present in a localised or disseminated form.

The localised form is confined to the upper respiratory region, appearing in approximately 25% of the patients (Bailey B., 2006)(Cummings C., 2005).

Up to 95% of patients will present with ear, nose and throat signs and symptoms:
- epistaxis
- sinusitis
- nasal disease
- hearing loss
- granular mucosa
- irregular mucosal thickening
- mucosal crusting (Gottschlich S., et. al., 2006), (Haris M., et. al., 2008).

Wegener's granulomatosis rhinologic symptoms are:
- nasal congestion with nasal obstruction
- anosmia
- crusting
- bloody rhinorrhea

The disease may progress to (Bailey B., 2006)(Cummings C., 2005):
- rhinitis
- sinusitis
- septal perforation
- painful or painless ulcers

- nasal airway stenosis
- saddle-nose deformity

Cannady *et al.* (2009) studied 120 patients with nasal signs and symptoms
- nasal crusts (69.2%)
- chronic sinusitis (60.8%)
- nasal obstruction (58.3%)
- bloody rhinorrhea (51.7%)
- septal perforation (32.5%)
- "saddle nose" deformity (22.7%) (Cannady SB., et. al., 2009).

Septal perforations were also common, Jennings *et al.* (1998) reporting 3 of 49 (6%) patients studied (Jennings CR, et. al., 1998), and "saddle nose" deformity is described in 10–25% of patients with nasal involvement (Cannady SB., et. al., 2009) (McDonald TJ, DeRemee RA., 1983) (McDonald TJ, et. al., 1974).

Nasal signs and symptoms are represented by nasal crusting, ulceration, and, in advanced cases due to septal destruction appears the saddle nose (Leavitt RY, Fauci AS., 1992) (Murty GE., 1990).

Nasal endoscopy assesses:
- edema
- crusting
- septal perforation
- mucosal cobblestoning (Tami TA, 2005)

Less common symptoms are (Bailey B., 2006)(Cummings C., 2005):
- hoarseness
- stridor (subglottic stenosis)

- painful or painless ulcers in oral cavities
- otalgia
- otorrhea
- conductive and sensorineural hearing loss
- uveitis
- scleritis
- episcleritis
- conjunctivitis

Otologic signs and symptoms vary:
- serous otitis media
- chronic otitis media
- sensorineural hearing loss
- vertigo
- tinnitus
- facial palsy (Pires APBA, et. al., 2008) (Cahali S, et. al., 1997).

As a first symptom and sign an otologic manifestations appear in 20 to 60% of cases of Wegener's granulomatosis (Pires APBA, et. al., 2008) (Rezende CEB, et. al., 2003) (Cahali S, et. al., 1997).

Ear involvement may occur in 20–70% of cases (Jennings CR, et. al., 1998) (McDonald TJ, et. al., 1974), most frequently encountered being external otitis secondary to chronic otitis media.

The middle ear is affected in 40–70% of cases (Jennings CR, et. al., 1998) (Vartiainen E, Nuutinen J., 1992).

Serous otitis media due to Eustachian tube dysfunction is the most common otological manifestation (Bradley PJ., 1983)(Parra-García GD., et. al., 2012)(Pereira DB, et. al., 2006) followed by chronic suppurative otitis media (24% of cases), mastoiditis and even facial nerve palsy (8–10% of cases) (Vartiainen E, Nuutinen J. H., 1992)(Takagi D., et. al., 2002).

Otological signs and symptoms are represented by the following diseases serous otitis media and supurative otitis media (Murty GE., 1990).

Lower limbs papulonecrotic lesions represent the most common skin injuries (Chung L, et. al., 2008) (Emedicine.Medscape.com [Internet]. Dermatologic manifestations of Wegener granulomatosis, Inc.; c2011 [updated 2013 Oct 23; cited 2014 Jan 29]).

Renal diseases are more frequently (75% to 80% of patients) classified as
- focal and segmental necrotizing glomerulonephritis
- generalized glomerulonephritis
- renal vasculitis (Cox NH, et. al., 2010) (Jennette JC, et. al., 2013) (Fernandes NC, et. al., 1998)

Disseminated form with pulmonary involvement is characterized by (Bailey B., 2006)(Cummings C., 2005):
- cough
- haemoptysis
- dyspnoea
- pleuritic pain

Systemic symptoms are unspecific (Bailey B., 2006)(Cummings C., 2005):
- night sweats
- weakness

- loss of appetite
- fever
- fatigue
- weight loss
- arthralgias

Most of the patients (95%) present nasal symptoms, being the first manifestation signs and symptoms. Lower respiratory tract (pulmonary) involvement without upper respiratory tract (nasal) symptoms or signs are unusual (Bailey B., 2006)(Cummings C., 2005). Renal involvement, even if it is subclinical, appears in the majority of cases.

There are 3 types of Wegener's granulomatosis based on clinical signs and symptoms (Cummings C., 2010)(Leavitt RY et al., 1990):

Wegener's granulomatosis **Type 1**:
- limited form of the disease
- upper airway symptoms (nasal)
    - nasal pain
    - bloody rhinorrhea
    - crusting
- few systemic findings

Wegener's granulomatosis **Type 2**:
- systemic symptoms and signs
- prolonged upper respiratory tract pseudoinfection:
    - continuous nasal discharge
    - nasal pain and tenderness
    - bloody rhinorrhea

- o ulceration
- o crusting
- lower airway symptoms (pulmonary)
  - o cough
  - o hemoptysis
  - o cavitary lesions on radiologic exam

Wegener's granulomatosis **Type 3**:
- systemic disease widely disseminated
- upper and lower airway involvement
- cutaneous lesions
- renal involvement

Due to the nonspecific signs and symptoms of Wegener's granulomatosis, the diagnosis and treatment may be delayed (Cummings C., 2010).

Until 1966 Wegener's granulomatosis was diagnosed with the classic triad (upper airway, pulmonary and renal involvement). In 1966 Carrington & Liebow (Carrington CB, Liebow., 1966)(Daggett RB. et.al., 1990) reported for the first time the limited forms of Wegener's granulomatosis.

In 1976 DeRemee proposed the "ELK" classification (DeRemee RA, et. al., 1976) (DeRemee RA, et. al., 1980), assessing the extent of the organ system involvement:
- "E" stands for ear, nose and throat involvement;
- "L" for lung involvement; and
- "K" for kidney involvement.

Laboratory and paraclinical diagnosis should involve
- complete blood cell count
- chemistry group
- urinalysis
- anticyto-plasmatic autoantibodies (ACPA) test
- rheumatoid factor
- chest radiograph

In limited forms it might be encountered:
- a mild anemia
- minimal elevation of the erythrocyte sedimentation rate (30–50/h)
- normal serum creatinine
- urinalysis
- normal aspect on chest radiograph

In the more severe forms it might be encountered:
- multiple lung cavity lesions
- renal involvement (nonspecific glomerulo-nephritis)
- abnormal urinary sediment
- elevated serum creatinine levels
- highly elevated erythrocyte sedimentation rate (above 100 mm/h)
- marked anemia
- very high titter ACPA test.

The most important factor in the diagnosis is represented by the nasal biopsy with a mucosal and submucosal non-specific inflammation with extensive necrosis and ulceration. As well, it might be encountered a predominantly epithelioid necrotizing granulomas and vasculitis interesting small arteries and veins.

Especially in young patients Wegener's granulomatosis symptoms might be misinterpreted as mild and persistent respiratory tract infectious disease (Stegmayr BG., et. al., 2000).

In table 1 there are exposed nasal granulomatosis lesions. Histopathologic exam is essential in establishing the diagnosis of granulomatosis disease (McDonald TJ., 1990).

Table 1. Granulomatosis diseases of the nose.

Bacterial etiology	**Fungal etiology**	**Unspecified etiology**
Rhinoscleroma	Rhinosporidiosis	Wegener's granulomatosis
Syphilis	Aspergillosis	Mediofacial malignant granuloma
Tuberculosis	Mucormycosis	Sarcoidosis
Lupus	Candidosis	
Leprosy	Blastomycosis	

Ophthalmic diseases which may appear are: conjunctivitis, episcleritis, uveitis and scleritis (Murty GE., 1990).

Upper respiratory tract involvement appears in approximately 75–93% of patients, and lower respiratory tract (pulmonary) involvement in 60–85% of patients (Holle JU., et. al., 2010). Other authors reported the impairment of the respiratory mucosa from the lower to the upper airways to appear in 15%–55% of the patients with Wegener's granulomatosis (Daum TE., et. al., 1995)(Gluth MB., et. al., 2003)(Hoffman GS., et. al., 2003)(Cordier JF., et. al., 1990). In approximately 25% of cases airways affection may be the only signs or symptoms (Lee AS., et. al., 2006).

Airway and pulmonary complications of Wegener's granulomatosis include:
- subglottic stenosis
- tracheal and bronchial inflammation
- tracheal and bronchial and stenoses
- granulomatous pulmonary nodules
- alveolar and cavitary infiltrates (Arcasoy SM, Kreit JW., 1999).

Upper airway tract manifestation are related to subglottic stenosis, which is not uncommon (Bevelaqua F., et. al., 1989)(Mokoka MC., et. al., 2013). In Wegener's granulomatosis subglottic stenosis being a life-threatening condition appears more frequently in younger patients than in multiorgan affected patients (Fauci AS., et. al., 1983) (Lebovics RS., et. al., 1992). In some cases there was necessary to perform a tracheostomy. The most affected are females (Hoffman GS., et. al., 2003) (Alaani A., et. al., 2004). Subglottic stenosis is a common found manifestation (Polychronopoulos VS., et. al., 2007) (Langford CA, 1996)(Screaton NJ., 1998).

Expiratory dyspnoea and stridor represents the most common presenting signs and symptoms (81.5% and 29.6%, respectively), but the patients may be asymptomatic depending on narrowing degree (Gluth MB, et. al., 2003).

Subglottic stenosis may occur during the quiescent phase due to maturation of subglottic scarring (Summers RM, et. al., 2002).

In our case series there was not necessary to perform a trachestomy. Subglottic stenosis may appear in 7–23% of cases, and as a presenting signs and symptoms may appear in only 1–6% of cases (Langford CA., et. al. 1996)(Solans-Laqué R., et. al., 2008)(Hernández-Rodríguez J., et. al., 2010).

Subglottic stenosis appears as a result of circumferential inflammation, edema, and fibrosis which extend for 3 to 4 cm below the vocal cords. Subglottic region is particularly susceptible to symptomatic narrowing due to cricoid cartilage complete ring. In the tracheal inferior part segment the symptoms are more easily tolerated due to the tracheal soft fibromembranous posterior wall.

Upper and lower respiratory tract endoscopy helps in the diagnosis and follow-up (Polychronopoulos VS., et. al., 2007).

In a study Fauci et al. (1983) have reported endobronchial abnormalities in 12 (15%) of 80 patients with Wegener's granulomatosis and lower respiratory tract affection, while Cordier et al. (1990) have reported the same sings and symptoms and/or hemorrhage in 41 (55%) of 74 patients.

Diagnosis

Presence of its triad
- necrotizing granulomatous inflammation of the respiratory tract,
- cutaneous necrotizing vasculitis
- glomerulonephritis

are characteristic for diagnosis (Cox NH, et. al., 2010) (Chung L, et. al., 2008).

Wegener's granulomatosis diagnosis is established based on:
- nasal biopsies with histopathologic examination
- chest x-ray (lower respiratory tract involvement)
- urine analysis (kidney involvement)
- cytoplasmic antineutrophilic cytoplasmic antibody (c-ANCA) test
- proteinase 3 (PR3) ANCA
- myeloperoxidase (MPO) ANCA
- C-reactive protein (CRP)
- hemoleucogram
- erythrocytes sedimentation rate (Briedigkeit L., et. al., 1993) (Holle JU., et. al., 2011) (Hilhorst M., et. al., 2013).

During the acute phase of Wegener's granulomatosis, titres of antineutrophil cytoplasmic antibodies (C-ANCA) are elevated. In initial phase they are elevated in 50% of patients and in general phase they are elevated in 95% of patients (Cummings C., 2010).

The c-ANCA (cytoplasmic immunofluorescence pattern) are highly specific and sensitive to Wegener's granulomatosis. Proteinase 3-ANCA (PR 3-ANCA,c-ANCA) and myeloperoxidase-ANCA (MPO-ANCA, p-ANCA) can activate neutrophils determining their adhesion to endothelial cells, releasing reactive oxygen species and lytic enzymes with the effect of vessel walls damage.

In Wegener's granulomatosis T regulatory lymphocytes CD4+CD25+FoxP3+Treg number and function were decreased, and an increased proportion of Treg lymphocytes was associated with more rapid remission (Morgan MD., et al., 2010).

Approximately 25–40% of patients, mainly with a limited form of Wegener's granulomatosis have undetectable serum levels of ANCA (Solans-Laqué R, et. al., 2008)(Finkielman JD., et al., 2007).

The c-ANCA test is highly sensitive for Wegener's granulomatosis, but a negative result does not exclude the diagnosis (Specks U. et. al., 1989)(Kallenberg CGM, 1990)(McDonald TJ., 1993). The c-ANCA titre may be used for Wegener's granulomatosis activity monitoring.

Davies, in 1982, and Van der Woude, in 1985, showed anti-neutrophil cytoplasmic antibodies of cytoplasmic pattern (C-ANCA), in GP, with a disease specificity of 99.3% (Brandt HR, et. al., 2009).

Originally ANCA antibodies are associated with necrotizing vasculitis, being classified to its stimulating antigen (Jennette JC, et. al., 2013) (Brandt HR, et. al., 2009):

- specific pattern for protein myeloperoxidase (MPO-ANCA) of perinuclear presentation (p-ANCA)
- specific pattern for proteinase 3 (PR3-ANCA) of cytoplasmic display (c-ANCA).

The biopsy is essential in establishment of the diagnosis. Sometimes in not specific revealing a nonspecific chronic inflammation associated with necrosis.

The biopsy should be taken from the involved organ (Bailey B., 2006)(Cummings C., 2005):
- nasal mucosa (turbinates, septum)
- lung, kidney
- skin

Abnormal laboratory values (Bailey B., 2006)(Cummings C., 2005):
- erythrocyte sedimentation rate
- haemoglobin
- serum creatinine
- culture (necessary to rule out granulomatous infectious agents: fungi, mycobacteria)
- serum c-ANCA
- ANCAs for anti-PR3 and ANCAs for antimyeloperoxidase (Erickson VR, Hwang PH, 2007)

Chest X ray and pulmonary CT scan may reveal bilateral nodules and cavitating infiltrations.

We describe 4 patients with Wegener's granulomatosis. One patient presented a prolonged evolution for more than 10 years in a stable condition.

The patients were hospitalized in ENT Department and Department of Medical Semiology I Timisoara, "Victor Babes" University of Medicine and Pharmacy Timisoara, Romania and followed for a period of 10 years. We analysed the patients files. One case is under control, the other 3 patients deceased.

Standard ENT exam was followed by a rigid and flexible endoscopic examination with DVD recording.

We used for the nasal endoscopic exam a 0 and 30°, 4 mm, rigid Karl Storz nasal endoscope (Figure 1) and flexible fiberlaryngoscope Karl-Storz Germany 1 100 1 RD 1 CE 0123 (Figure 2). For laryngeal endoscopic exam we used a 70°, rigid Karl Storz laryngoscope endoscope (Figure 3).

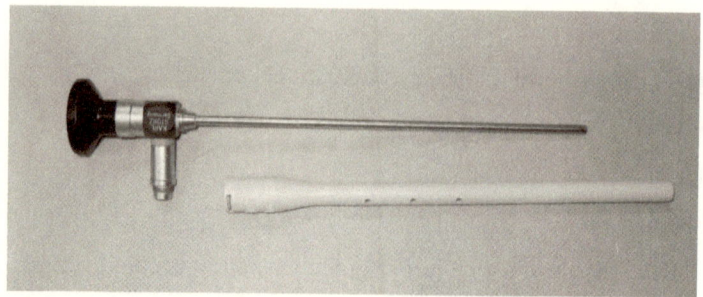

Figure 1. 0°, 4 mm, rigid Karl Storz nasal endoscope.

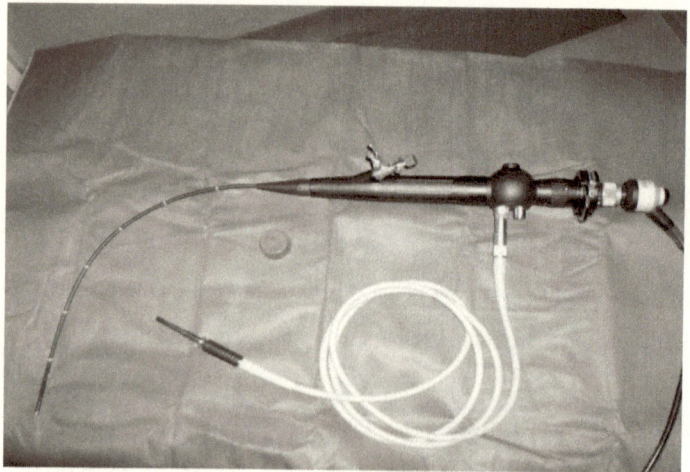

Figure 2. Flexible fiberlaryngoscope Karl-Storz Germany 1 100 1 RD 1 CE 0123.

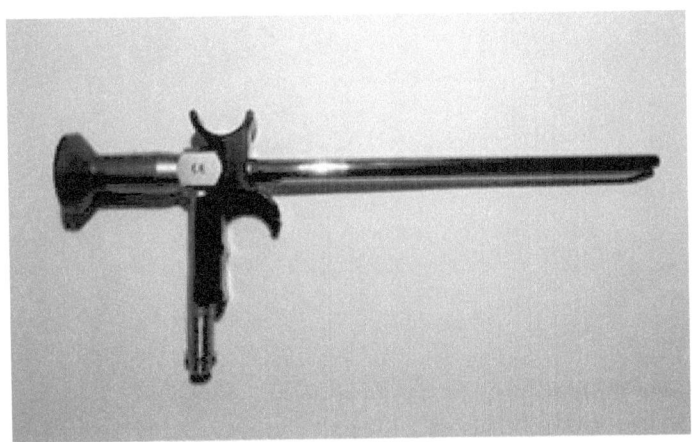

Figure 3. 70°, rigid Karl Storz laryngoscope endoscope.

The images were digitally acquired with a Stryker Endoscopy 597T Medical Video Camera (Figure 4), a light source STORZ (Karl-Storz) Xenon Nova **20**1315 20 (Figure 5), a videorecorder S-VHS Panasonic NV-SD230 (Figure 6), in .jpeg format with MediLive ImageBox Zeiss (Figure 7) and with DVD recorder Panasonic DMR-ES10 (Figure 8). In figure 9 there are instruments used for nasal biopsies and endoscopic nasal and sinus surgery.

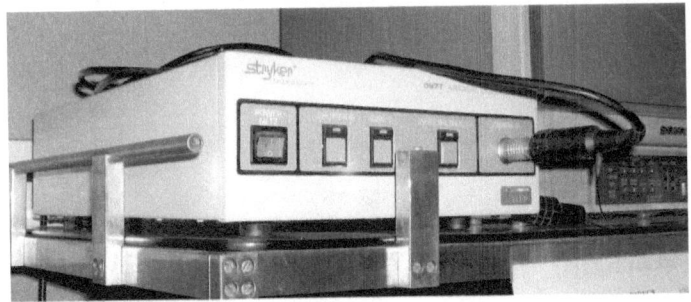

Figure 4. Stryker Endoscopy 597T Medical Video Camera

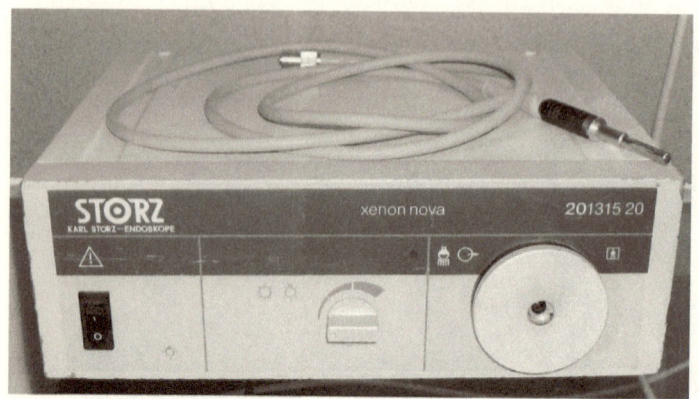

Figure 5. Light source STORZ (Karl-Storz) Xenon Nova 201315 20

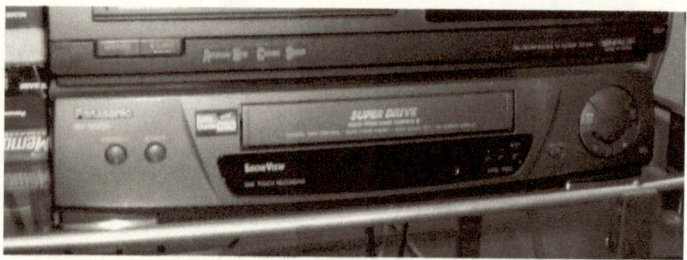

Figure 6. Videorecorder S-VHS Panasonic NV-SD230.

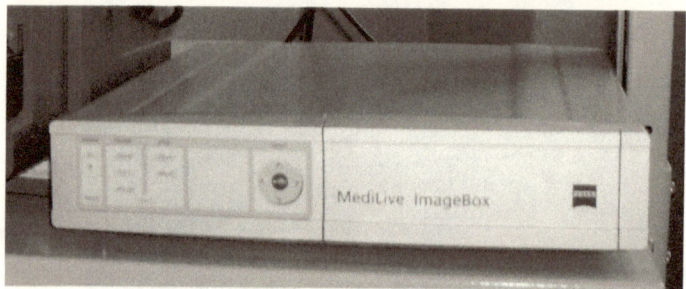

Figure 7. MediLive ImageBox Zeiss.

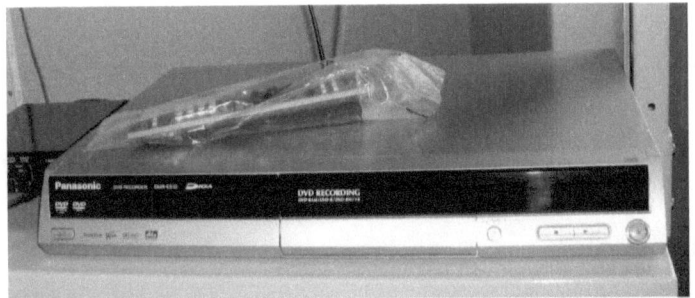

Figure 8. DVD recorder Panasonic DMR-ES10.

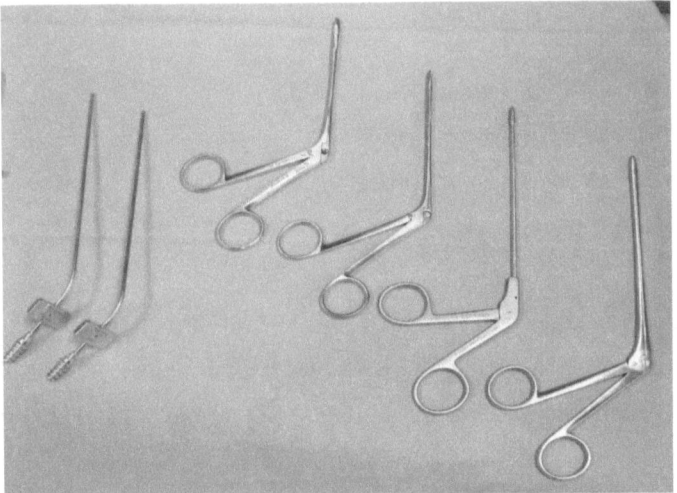

Figure 9. Instruments for nasal biopsy and endoscopic nasal and sinus surgery.

Case No. 1

Female patient, I.Z., 27-year-old, was admitted in ENT Department Timisoara and 3rd Clinic of Internal Medicine with the following signs and symptoms:
- left frontal headache
- bilateral nasal obstruction
- bilateral mucopurulent rhinorrhea
- anosmia
- recurrent epistaxis
- bilateral hearing loss

Personal pathological antecedents revealed:
- left chronic maxillary sinusitis
- secondary anemia

Standard ENT exam was followed by a rigid and flexible endoscopic examination using a 0°, 4 mm, rigid Karl Storz nasal endoscope and flexible fiberlaryngoscope Karl-Storz Germany 1 100 1 RD 1 CE 0123. For laryngeal endoscopic exam we used a 70°, rigid Karl Storz laryngoscope endoscope.

Nasal rigid endoscopy revealed a bilateral pituitary involvement by a granulomatous inflammatory process, hemorrhagic crusts and granulation tissue and a septal ulceration (Figure 10, Figure 11, Figure 12, Figure 13 and Figure 14).

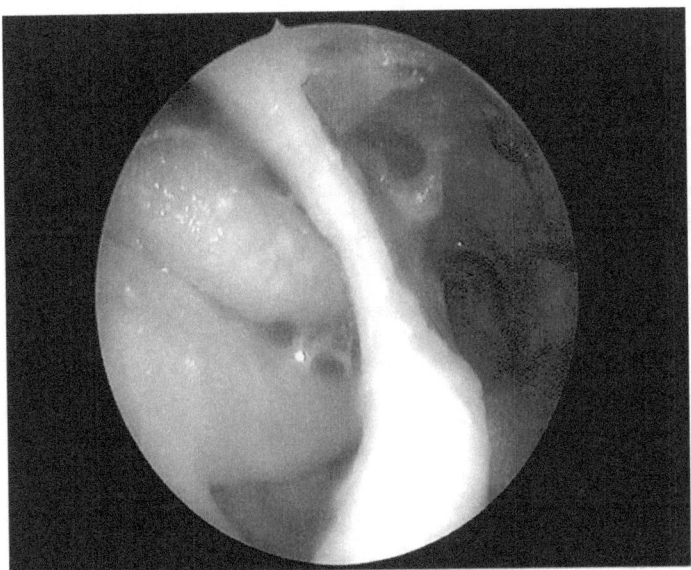

Figure 10. Nasal rigid endoscopic exam using a 0°, 4 mm, rigid Karl Storz nasal endoscope assesses the septal perforation.

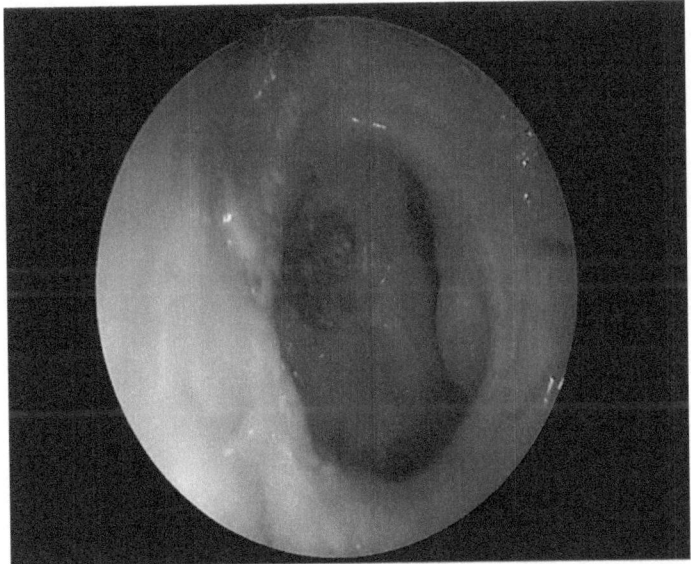

Figure 11. Nasal rigid endoscopic exam reveals choane and rhinopharyngeal crusts.

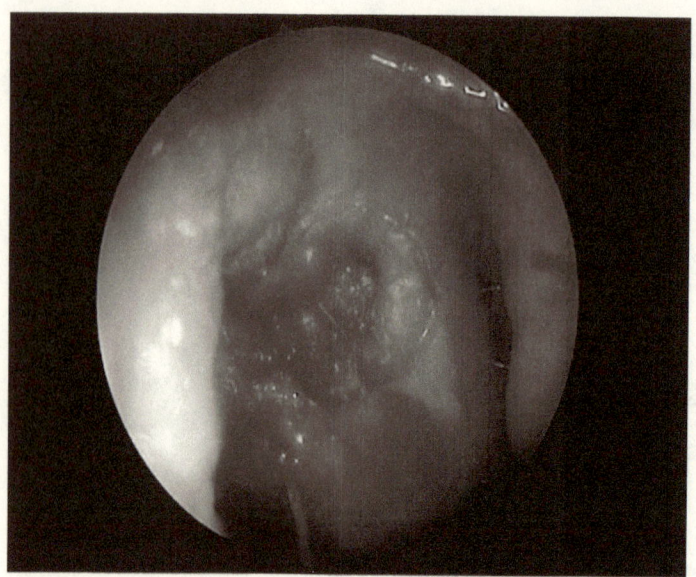

Figure 12. Nasal rigid endoscopic – detail on rhinopharyngeal crusts and granulomatous inflammatory process.

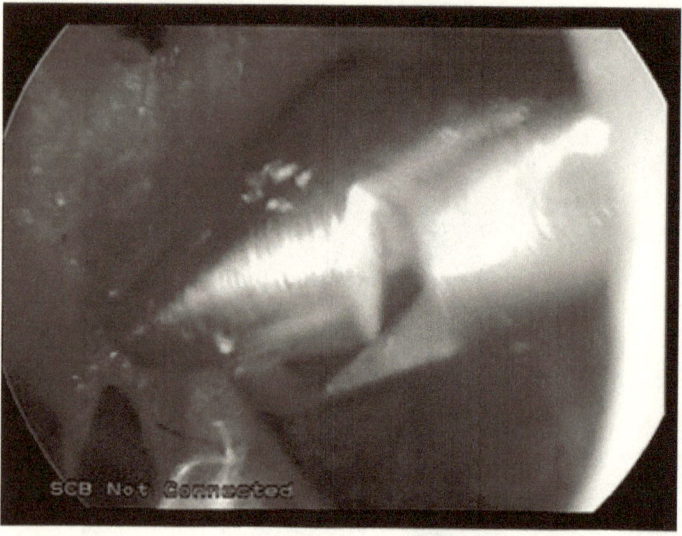

Figure 13. Nasal rigid endoscopy – a biopsy forceps was used for septal ulceration biopsy.

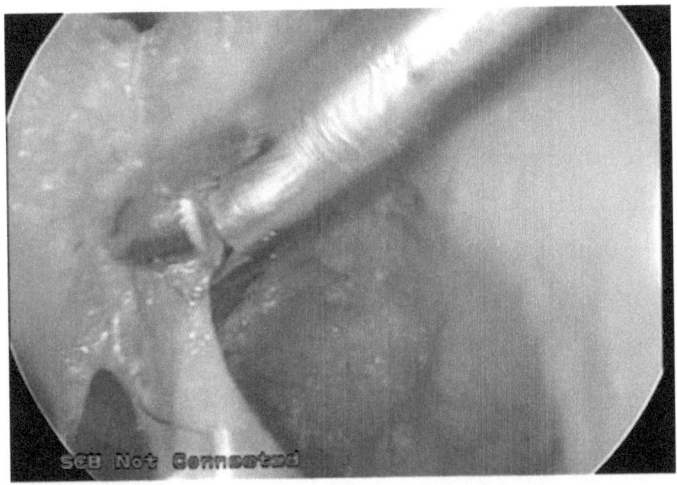

Figure 14. Nasal rigid endoscopy – a biopsy forceps was used for septal ulceration biopsy (granulomatous tissue).

The endoscopic exam was performed in local anesthesia with/or without intravenous sedation. All visible nasal hemorrhagic crusts were removed, followed by cleaning of the septum, nasal floor, and turbinates tissues in order to provide enough bioptic material for an accurate diagnosis.

The histopathological exam assessed a granulomatosis inflammatory process, with extensive fibrinoid necrotic zones and necrotic epitheloid granulomas.

Paraclinic and laboratory analysis revealed:
- erythrocyte sedimentation rate (ESR) 103 mm/h
- haemoglobin (Hb) 8.6 mg%
- hematocrit (Ht) 28.6%
- blood urea 17mg%
- serum creatinine 1 mg%
- ACPA test with high level of anticytoplasmatic autoantibodies
- chest radiography – normal X-ray image

Internal medicine exam revealed a segmental and focal chronic glomerulonephritis. Wegener's granulomatosis diagnosis has been established based on ENT clinic, endoscopic and internal medicine exams in conjunction with laboratory, paraclinic and histopathological exams.

Histopathological exam were performed on biopsy specimen.

Seriate micro sections at 5 μ were performed according to usual histological techniques. Two sections were stained with Hematoxylin-Eosin in order to establish histological and grading diagnosis.

Histopathological exam assessed a necrotising granulomatous vasculitis which interested small arteries and venules, with Langhans' giant cells, neutrophil infiltration of the same vessels and fibrinoid necrosis.

Case No. 2

Female patient, S.M., 25-year-old, was admitted in ENT Department Timisoara and 3rd Clinic of Internal Medicine with the following signs and symptoms:
- bilateral chemosis
- nasal obstruction
- mild dyspnea
- headache
- anosmia

Personal pathological antecedents revealed:
- bronchial asthma diagnosed 3 years ago

Standard ENT exam was followed by a rigid and flexible endoscopic examination using a 0°, 4 mm, rigid Karl Storz nasal endoscope and flexible fiberlaryngoscope Karl-Storz Germany 1 100 1 RD 1 CE 0123. For laryngeal endoscopic exam we used a 70°, rigid Karl Storz laryngoscope endoscope.

Nasal rigid endoscopy revealed bloody crusts covering nasal mucosa (Figure 15) and a nasal septum cartilage perforation. Laryngeal 70° endoscopic exam revealed a subglottic stenosis which determined the mild dyspnea (Figure 16). During hospitalization, the dyspnea has aggravated, especially being inspiratory.

Under local anaesthesia we performed a nasal biopsy with histopathological exam. The patient was addressed to a dermatologic exam with a subsequent biopsy exam from elbows and knees petechial cutaneous lesions.

Nasal biopsy histopathological exam revealed a mucosal and submucosal non-specific inflammatory process.

Cutaneous biopsy histopathological exam revealed the same non-specific inflammatory process.

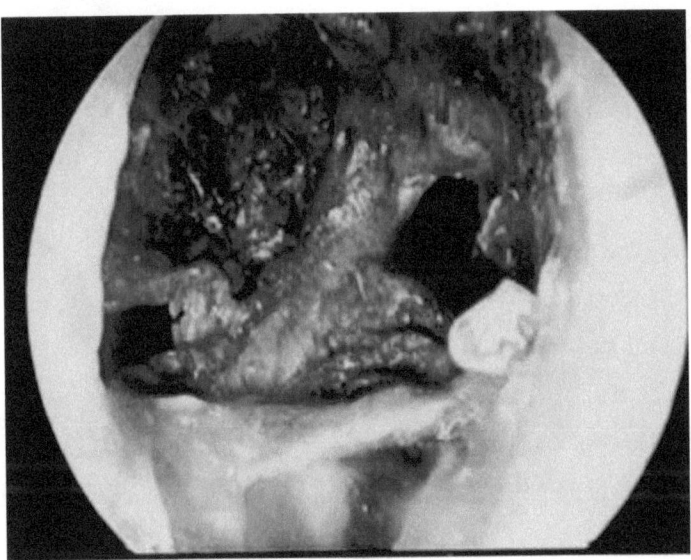

Figure 15. 0° nasal rigid endoscopic exam revealing in left nasal fossa in posterior 1/3, anterior to the left choanae, bloody crusts covering nasal mucosa.

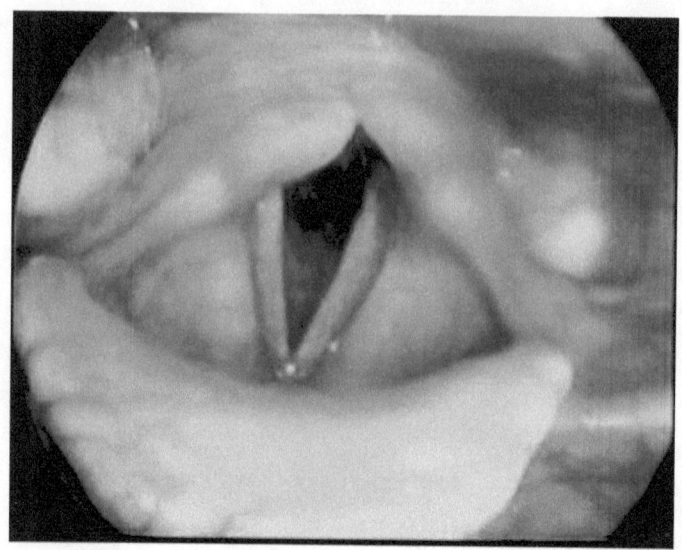

Figure 16. Laryngeal 70°, rigid endoscopic exam revealed a subglottic stenosis. Normal aspect of the glottic and supraglottic levels.

Laboratory and paraclinic exams showed:
- ESR 120 mm/h
- Hb 8.2 mg%
- Ht 27.4%
- high level of anticytoplasmic autoantibodies on ACPA test
- chest radiography – multiple cavitary and non-cavitary nodules in both lungs

Internal medicine exam revealed a focal chronic glomerulonephritis and ophthalmologic exam a bilateral episcleritis.

Case No. 3

Male patient, N.P., of 52-year-old, was admitted in ENT Department Timisoara and 3rd Clinic of Internal Medicine with the following signs and symptoms:
- bilateral nasal obstruction
- oral breathing
- bilateral mucopurulent rhinorrhea
- headache
- asthenia
- severe malaise

The general clinical exam was under normal limits.

Nasal endoscopic exam with a 0° rigid endoscope reveled:
- nasal mucosa congested and swollen
- nasal mucosa covered with bloody crusts
- nasal mucosa ulceration

The nasal endoscopic exam was followed by a nasal biopsy with a histopathological exam which assessed:
- chronic inflam-matory granulomatosis process with
- extended areas of suppurative necrosis

Laboratory and paraclinical exam:
- ESR 116 mm/h
- Hb 10.7%
- serum creatinine 2.1 mg%
- high level of anticytoplasmic autoantibodies on ACPA test

Case No. 4

Female patient, Z.I., 27-year-old, was admitted into Nephrology Department with the following diagnosis:
- ANCA positive vasculitis
- Chronic secondary glomerulonephritis
- Nephritic syndrome
- Urinary infection with *Klebsiella*
- Mild secondary anemia
- Respiratory insufficiency
- Bilateral supurative otitis media

Because the patient presented a respiratory insufficiency and a bilateral supurative otitis media she was addressed to ENT Department.

ENT clinic and endoscopic exam revealed the following diagnosis:
- Subglottic stenosis
- Bilateral supurative otitis media
- Chronic nasal inflammatory granulomatous process
- Left maxillary and frontal sinusitis

Laryngeal 70°, rigid endoscopic exam revealed a subglottic stenosis, with a normal aspect of the glottic and supraglottic levels (Figure 17).

We performed a nasal endoscopic biopsy which revealed the diagnosis of Wegener's granulomatosis.

Laboratory and paraclinical exams:
- ESR 91 mm/h
- Hb 8.58%
- serum creatinine 2.6 mg%
- high level of anticytoplasmic autoantibodies on ACPA test
- anti-MPO (myeloperoxidase antibody) was negative
- anti-PR3 (proteinase 3) was positive
- chest X-ray was in normal limits

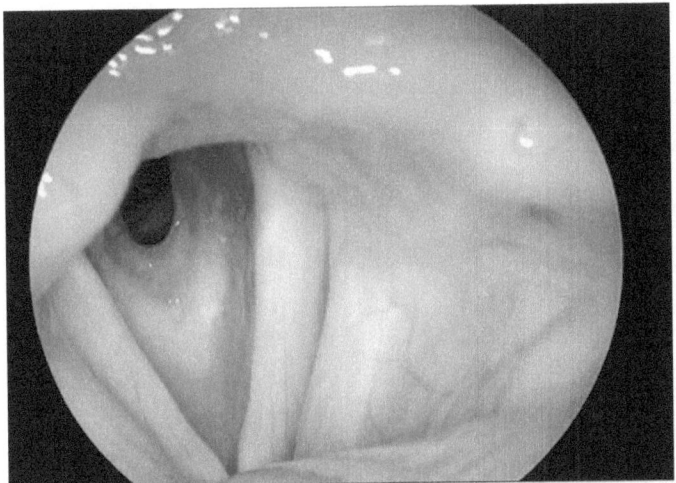

Figure 17. Laryngeal 70°, rigid endoscopic exam revealed a subglottic stenosis. Normal aspect of the glottic and supraglottic levels.

Differential diagnosis

Wegener's granulomatosis must be differentiated from other causes of granulomatous rhinosinusitis, infections and vasculitis, such as:
- traumatic granulomas
- cocaine-induced lesions
- bacterial and fungal infections
- microscopic polyangiitis
- other vasculitis

Granulomatosis diseases of the nose include (McDonald TJ., 1990):
- bacterial infections
    - rhinoscleroma
    - tuberculosis
    - syphilis
    - lupus
    - leprosy
- fungal infections
    - rhinosporidiosis
    - aspergillosis
    - mucormycosis
    - candidosis
    - histoplasmosis
    - blastomycosis
- diseases with unspecified etiology
    - Wegener's granulomatosis
    - mediofacial malignant granuloma
    - sarcoidosis).

Wegener's granulomatosis otologic manifestations differential diagnosis includes:
- tuberculous otitis media
- cholesteatoma
- Langerhans cell histiocytosis
- neoplastic diseases
- other forms of vasculitis
- sarcoidosis
- systemic lupus erythematosus

Subglottic stenosis differential diagnosis implies the following diseases:
- post-intubation stenosis
- post-infectious stenosis
- tuberculosis
- diphtheria
- syphilis
- relapsing polychondritis
- chemical irritation
- obstruction by a foreign body (Langford CA, et. al., 1996)
- other systemic diseases
  - Crohn's disease
  - Sarcoidosis
  - Behcet's syndrome (Prince JS., et. al., 2002)(Hervier B., et. al., 2006).

Being a rare, autoimmune systemic disease, Wegener's granulomatosis, represents an important attention for ENT practitioners due to continuous evolution and multiorganic involvement. Disease onset is unspecific, with upper airway involvement, a "persistent cold", being difficult to differentiate it from a prolonged evolution common cold.

Pathology

Wegener's granulomatosis histopathological features include:
- medium and small vessels vasculitis
- intramural, eccentric, necrotizing granulomatous lesions
- microabscesses may appear

In Figures 18–23, there are the histopathologic exams performed with Hematoxylin–Eosin (HE) staining, Periodic Acid–Schiff (PAS) reaction and argentic staining (PASM, Periodic Acid–Silver Methenamine).

We pbserve the microscopic aspects of glomerulonephritis with loop necrosis, semilunar cells and fibrosis (20×), skin ulceration and striated muscle inflammatory reactions.

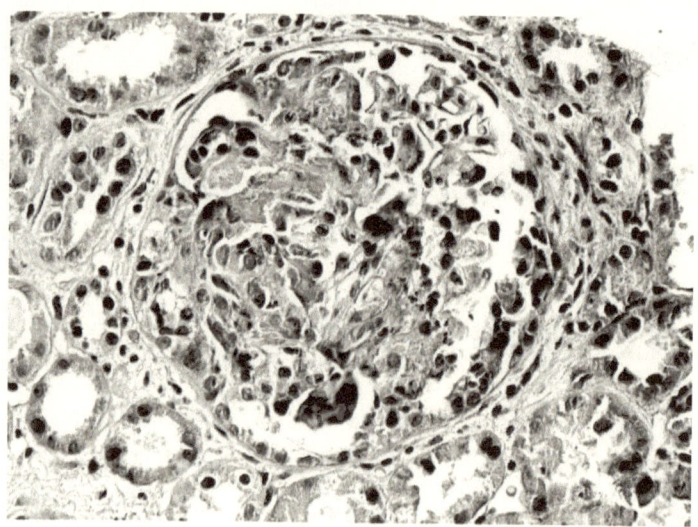

Figure 18. Glomerulonephritis with loop necrosis and semilunar cells. HE staining, ×200.

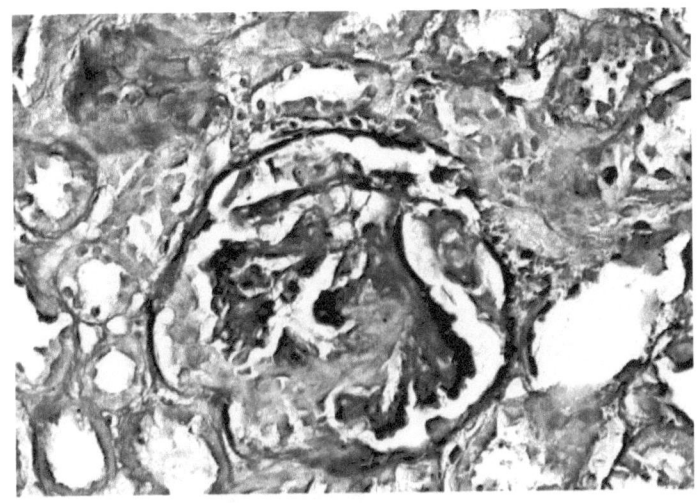

Figure 19. Glomerulonephritis with semilunar cells. PAS staining, ×200

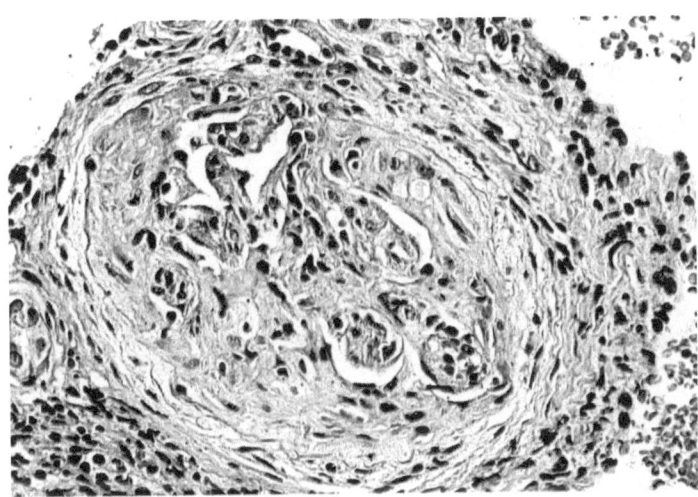

Figure 20. Glomerulonephritis with semilunar fibrosis. HE staining, ×200.

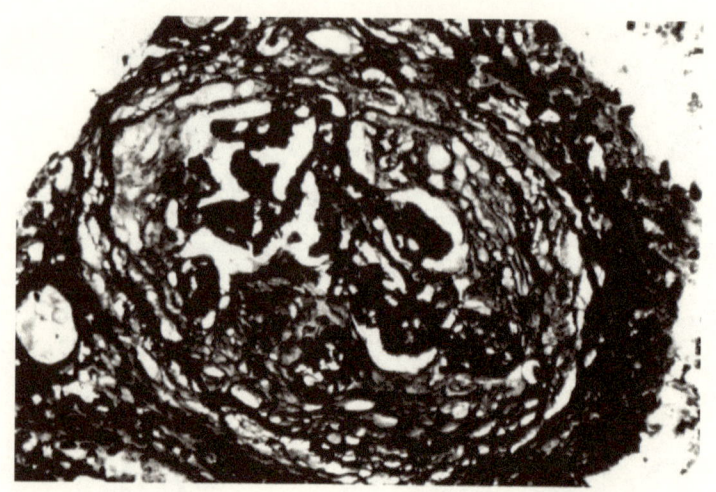

Figure 21. Glomerulonephritis with semilunar fibrosis. Argentic staining (PASM), ×200.

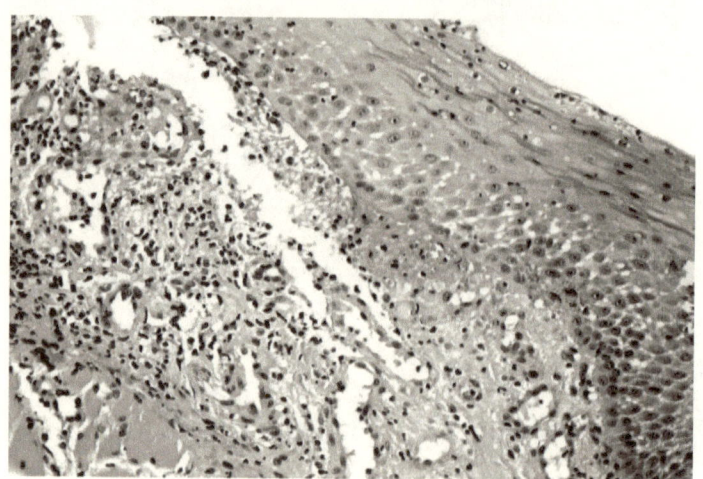

Figure 22. Skin ulceration. HE staining, ×200.

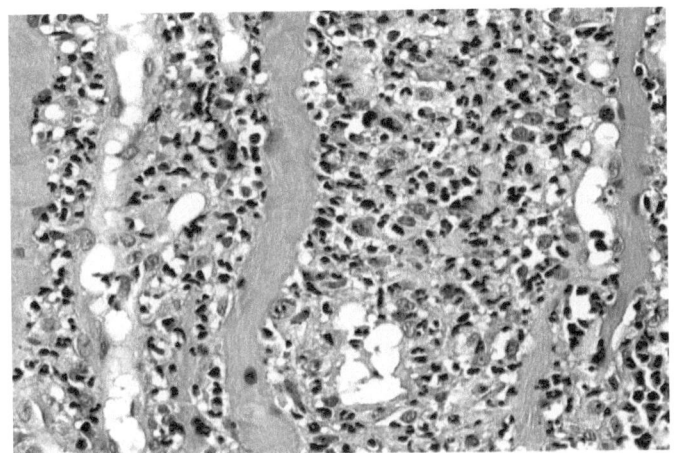

Figure 23. Striated muscle inflammatory reactions underneath the skin ulceration. HE staining, ×200.

Treatment

Being a multiorgan disease, Wegener's granulomatosis is treated by a multidisciplinary team of physicians, which include an otolaryngologist and internists, based on disease severity (Wung PK, Stone JH, 2006).

Immunosuppression is indicated in order to achieve remission, followed by dosages adjustment for remission maintenance, with the following agents:

- cyclophosphamide
    - oral administration – 2 mg/kg per day with a maximum dose of 200 mg/ day)
    - 6 months to 1 year
    - the dosage is tapered gradually with symptoms disappearance
    - it should be replaced, when remission is obtained, with less toxic agents such as methotrexate, azathioprine, or mycophenolate mofetil
- methotrexate
    - for Wegener's granulomatosis type 1
    - begins at 0.25 mg/kg/week, increased to maximum 25 mg/week
    - continued for 1 year
    - the dosage may be tapered, or stopped
- glucocorticoids
    - administered concurrently with cyclophosphamide or methotrexate
    - starting dose – prednisone 0.5 to 1.0 mg/kg/day up to a maximum of 80 mg/day (Wung PK, Stone JH, 2006)
    - for 1 month
    - dosage tapering is performed for 6 to 9 months

Treatment should be started as soon as possible (Takagi D, et. al., 2002).

Cyclophosphamide should be initiated in early stage, being a more advantageous than pulse doses, stage-adapted treatment, or Cyclosporin A (Briedigkeit L., et. al., 1993) (Takagi D., et. al., 2002) (Allen NB., et. al., 1993) (Briedigkeit L., et. al., 1993) (Reinhold-Keller E., et. al., 1993) (Reinhold-Keller E, et. al., 1994).

Other studies showed the advantages of steroid pulse therapy (Frascà GM., et. al., 1993) (Georganas C., et. al., 1996).

Unfortunately relapses are common in this disease, rituximab in combination with steroids, being considered safe and effective as an alternative to Cyclophosphamide (Bolton WK, Sturgill BC., 1998).

Immunosuppressive drugs are the first-line therapy (Rossini BAA, et. al., 2010) (Scalcon MRR, et. al. 2008) (Rezende CEB, et. al., 2003).

With corticosteroids and cyclophosphamide, Mc Donald and Remee assessed 411 cases, otaining a mean survival rate of 75% in 5.8 years (Dey A, et. al., 2008).

Antibiotics, mainly trimethoprim-sulfamethoxazole, should be administered for prophylaxis against *Pneumocystis jiroveci* (formerly *Pneumocystis carinii*) pneumonia (PCP), which may develop during immunosuppression and have a role in preventing recurrences (Regan MJ. et al., 2001).

Other therapeutic agents are indicated in resistant cases:
- rituximab (chimeric monoclonal antibody)(Sanchez-Cano D. et. al., 2008)
- mycophenolate mofetil – in patients who cannot be treated with cyclophosphamide (Stassen PM. et. al., 2007)

Sinonasal signs and symptoms are treated with:
- topical nasal steroids, nasal irrigations and nasal debridement
- lowdose systemic steroids
- antibiotics for bacterial infection (typically *Staphylococcus* species)

- surgical reconstruction for saddle nose deformity correction and septal perforation repair;
- FESS (functional endoscopic sinus surgery) for chronic nasal crusting

Early treatment of remission induction is crucial to reverse the renal affection, being performed, in the first 3 months of signs and symptoms, with corticosteroids and cyclophosphamide (Cox NH, et. al., 2010) (Chung L, et. al., 2008) (Brandt HR, et. al., 2009).

Actually the most studied treatment is rituximab, being reccomended by EULAR as an alternative drug for refractory disease, (dose of 375 mg/m²/week for 4 weeks) (Lutalo PM, D'Cruz DP., 2014).

Another remission alternative treatment is methotrexate 15-25 mg/ week combined with folic acid, maintenance may be performed with azathioprine 2 mg/kg/day; leflunomide 20-30 mg/day or rituximab 1g IV every 6 months for 2 years (Lutalo PM, D'Cruz DP., 2014).

Before starting the treatment of Wegener's granulomatosis a suspected infections and/or nasal carriage of *Staphylococcus aureus* should be taken into consideration (Faurschou M., et. al., 2013).

In approximately 90% of patients there may be observed a remission on conventional immunosuppressive therapy, but relapses are not uncommon (Fauci AS., et. al., 1983).

In the literature there are evidence regarding the role of trimethoprim-sulfamethoxazole in reducing the trigger factors which may exacerbate the Wegener's granulomatosis (Zycinska K., et. al., 2009).

There are evidence of other therapeutic agents in Wegener's granulomatosis treatment, such as rituximab, a monoclonal antibody against CD20 (B lymphocytes), especially indicated for remission induction and relapses prevention (Rhee EP., et. al., 2010).

In approximately 20–26% of patients the treatment ensured an improvement, while the rest of the patients may require local surgical treatment (Hernández-Rodríguez J., et. al., 2010).

Regarding subglottic stenosis an endoscopic dilatation, endoscopic laser excision or surgical resection may be performed ((Hernández-Rodríguez J., et. al., 2010) (Alaani A., et. al., 2004).

Langford et al. (1996) proposed a technique based on intralesional long-acting corticosteroid injection with promising results regarding subglottic stenosis (Solans-Laqué R,, et. al., 2008) (Wolter NE., et. al., 2010) (Rasmussen N., 2013).

Generally the subglottic stenosis is not influenced by immunosuppressive therapy, but endoscopic CO_2 laser treatment is an option (Strange C., 1990).

Mitomycin- C, an antifibroblastic agent may soak the stenotic area with a success rate of 85% in preventing restenosis (Arebro et al., 2012).

In case of subglottic stenosis systemic immunosuppressive therapy and manual dilation followed by with intralesional corticosteroids may prevent the necessity of tracheostomy. Laser resection may not be beneficial due to consecutive extensive scarring and stenosis (Lebovics RS, et. al., 1992).

Pulmonary fibrosis appears in patients with vasculitis mainly in active disease than in remission period (Bhanji A, Karim M., 2010), and occasionally is associated with Cyclophosphamide therapy (Hamada K., et. al., 2003).

Springer et al. (2014) assessed treatment length and its relationship with the relapse risk (52% of relapses appeared during off treatment interval. Regarding overall side effects or disease related morbidity, there were no differences between the short- and long-term therapeutic options (Adu D., et. al., 1997) (Clain JM., et. al. 2014) (Tomasson G., et. al., 2014).

Case No. 1

The patient was rehospitalized in the 3rd Clinic of Internal Medicine and started the treatment treatment with cyclophosphamide (2 mg/kg per day for 1 year, with a dose tapered gradually while symptoms remissions) and glucocorticoids (with a starting dose of prednisone 1.0 mg/kg/day for 1 month, and a dose tapering for the next 6 months).

In the first phase of the disease serum ANCA (anti-neutrophil cytoplasmic antibody) were increased, but under treatment we encountered normalization.

The disease did not relapse.

ENT clinic, endoscopic and internal medicine exams in conjunction with laboratory and paraclinic exams performed every 3 months revealed a stable condition without any complications.

Case No. 2

The patient followed an admission in 3rd Clinic of Internal Medicine and corticosteroid (administered concurrently with cyclophosphamide with an initiating dose of prednisone 0.5 mg/kg/day for 1 month followed by a dosage tapering for 9 months) and cyclophosphamide (oral administration, 2 mg/kg per day for 12 months, with a dosage tapering gradually with symptoms disappearance) treatment was initiated. Trimethoprim-sulfamethoxazole was administered for prophylaxis against pneumonia and in order to prevent symptoms and signs relapsing.

Unfortunately the serum ANCA was still at high levels. The patient underwent periodic urinanalyses and serum ANCA levels assessment.

The patient died 3 years later.

Case No. 3

The patient was admitted to Department of Nephrology. The following treatment was initiated:
- corticosteroid (administered concurrently with cyclophosphamide with an initiating dose of prednisone 0.5 mg/kg/day for 1 month followed by a dosage tapering for 9 months)
- cyclophosphamide (oral administration, 2 mg/kg per day for 12 months, with a dosage tapering gradually with symptoms disappearance)
- trimethoprim-sulfamethoxazole was administered for prophylaxis against pneumonia and in order to prevent symptoms and signs relapsing

Unfortunately the patient died after two years.

Case No. 4

In Nephrology Department the patient initiated the treatment as follows:
- corticosteroid (prednisone 0.5 mg/kg/day for 1 month followed by a dosage tapering for 6 months)
- cyclophosphamide (oral administration, 2 mg/kg per day for 12 months, with a dosage tapering gradually in accordance with symptoms
- trimethoprim-sulfamethoxazole for prophylaxis against pneumonia

The evolution was favourable.

Unfortunately the patient developed:
- Secondary arterial hypertension
- Iatrogenic secondary amenorrhea
- Segmental and focal chronic glomerulonephritis

The patient deceased 4 years later.

Prognosis

Most of the patients respond well to treatment. Long-term complications are chronic renal failure, hearing loss and deafness.

Disease prognosis is less favorable once the kidneys are affected (Briedigkeit L., et. al., 1993), but early detection and treatment initiation should improve the prognosis (Holle JU., et. al., 2011) (Hilhorst M., et. al., 2013).

Conclusions

Granulomatosis with polyangiitis (Wegener's granulomatosis) is a rare and a serious systemic vasculitis with preferential involvement of the upper and lower respiratory tract, eyes skin and kidneys.

The diagnosis is established based on the clinical and paraclinical exams.

Granulomatosis with polyangiitis may affect any airway segment, determining inflammation, ulceration, pseudomembranes, tracheobronchomalacia, cartilage destruction and laryngeal-tracheo-bronchial stenoses.

REFERENCES

- Adu D, Pall A, Luqmani RA, Richards NT, Howie AJ, Emery P, Michael J, Savage CO, Bacon PA. Controlled trial of pulse versus continuous prednisolone and cyclophosphamide in the treatment of systemic vasculitis. QJM, 1997, 90(6):401–409.
- Alaani A, Hogg RP, Drake Lee AB. Wegener's granulomatosis and subglottic stenosis: management of the airway. J Laryngol Otol 2004; 118: 786–790.
- Allen NB, Caldwell DS, Rice JR, McCallum RM. Cyclosporin A therapy for Wegener's granulomatosis. Adv Exp Med Biol, 1993, 336:473–476.
- Antunes T, Barbas CSV. Granulomatose de Wegener. J Bras Pneumol 2005;31(Suppl 1):S21–S26.
- Arcasoy SM, Kreit JW. Recurrent sinusitis, arthralgias, and progressive dyspnea in a 26 year old woman. Chest 1999;115(6):1731-4.
- Arebro J, Henriksson G, Macchiarini P, Juto JE. New treatment of subglottic stenosis due to Wegener's granulomatosis. Acta Otolaryngol 2012; 132: 995–1001. doi: 10.3109/00016489.2012.674213.
- Bailey B. Head and neck surgery – otolaryngology, 4th edn. Lippincott Williams & Wilkins, Philadelphia, Pa. 2006.
- Bevelaqua F, Schicchi JS, Haas F, Axen K, Levin N. Aortic arch anomaly presenting as exercise-induced asthma. Am Rev Respir Dis, 1989, 140(3):805–808.
- Bhanji A, Karim M. Pulmonary fibrosis – an uncommon mani-festation of anti-myeloperoxidase-positive systemic vasculitis? NDT Plus, 2010, 3(4):351–353.

- Bolton WK, Sturgill BC. Methylprednisolone therapy for acute crescentic rapidly progressive glomerulonephritis. Am J Nephrol, 1998, 9(5):368–375.
- Bradley PJ. Wegener's granulomatosis of the ear. J Laryngol Otol, 1983, 97(7):623–626.
- Brandt HR, Arnone M, Valente NY, Sotto MN, Criado PR. Medium and large vessel vasculitis. An Bras Dermatol. 2009;84:55-67.
- Briedigkeit L, Kettritz R, Göbel U, Natusch R. Prognostic factors in Wegener's granulomatosis. Postgrad Med J, 1993, 69(817):856–861.
- Briedigkeit L, Ulmer M, Göbel U, Natusch R, Reinhold-Keller E, Gross WL. Treatment of Wegener's granulomatosis. In: Gross WL (ed). ANCA-associated vasculitides: immunological and clinical aspects. Vol. 336, Advances in Experimental Medicine and Biology, 1993, 491–495.
- Cahali S, SouzaMMA, SilveiraMC, CabaliMB, Cahali RB.Wegener's granulomatosis—case report with otological manifestation as first symptom. Braz J Otorhinolaryngol 1997;63(1):72–74.
- Cannady SB, Batra PS, Koening C, Lorenz RR, Citardi MJ, Langford C, Hoffman GS. Sinonasal Wegener granuloma-tosis: a single-institution experience with 120 cases. Laryn-goscope, 2009, 119(4):757–761.
- Carrington CB, Liebow AA. Limited forms of angitis and granulomatosis of Wegener's type. Am J Med, 1966, 41(4): 497–527.
- Chung L, Kea B, Fiorentino D. Cutaneous vasculitis. In: Bolognia J, Jorizzo J, Rapini R, and editors. Dermatology. New York: Elsevier, 2008. p.360-61.
- Clain JM, Cartin-Ceba R, Fervenza FC, Specks U. Experience with rituximab in the treatment of antineutrophil cytoplasmic antibody associated vasculitis. Ther Adv Musculoskelet Dis, 2014, 6(2):58–74.
- Cordier JF, Valeyre D, Guillevin L, Loire R, Brechot JM. Pulmonary Wegener's granulomatosis. A clinical and imaging study of 77 cases. Chest 1990; 97(4):906–12.

- Correa JC, Azevedo AG, Rubens J, Rocha G. Granulomatose de Wegener: análise de dois casos. J Bras Med 1985;48(6): 34–38.
- Cotch MF, Hoffman GS, Yerg DE, et al: The epidemiology of Wegener's granulomatosis: estimates of the five-year period prevalence, annual mortality, and geographic disease distribution from population-based data sources. Arthritis Rheum 1996; 39:87–92.
- Cox NH, Jorizzo JL, Bourke JF, Savage COS. Vasculitis, neutrophilic dermatoses and related disorders. In: Burns T, Breathnach S, Cox N, Griffiths C, editors. Rook's textbook of dermatology. London: Wiley Blackwell; 2010. p. 2417-19.
- Cummings C. Otolaryngology: head and neck surgery, 4th edn. Mosby, New York, 2005.
- Daggett RB, Haghighi P, Terkeltaub RA. Nasal cocaine abuse causing an aggressive midline intranasal and pharyngeal destructive process mimicking midline reticulosis and limited Wegener's granulomatosis. J Rheumatol, 1990, 17(6):838–840.
- Daum TE, Specks U, Colby TV, Edell ES, Brutinel MW, Prakash UB et al. Tracheobronchial involvement in Wegener's granulomatosis. Am J Respir Crit Care Med 1995; 151(2 Pt 1):522–6.
- DeRemee RA, McDonald TJ, Harrison EG Jr, Coles DT. Wegener's granulomatosis. Anatomic correlates, a proposed classification. Mayo Clin Proc, 1976, 51(12):777–781.
- DeRemee RA, McDonald TJ, Weiland LH. Wegener's granulomatosis, polymorphic reticulosis, and lymphomatoid granulomatosis: a comparative analysis in sarcoidosis and other granulomatous diseases. Proceedings of the 8th Inter-national Conference on Sarcoidosis and Other Granulomatous Diseases, United Kingdom, Alpha Omega Publishing, 1980, 738–742.

- Dey A, Arunabha DC, Sudipta P, Susmita K, Mita S. A young lady presented with limited pulmonary Weneger's Granulomatosis. Lung India. 2008;25:168-71.
- Emedicine.Medscape.com [Internet]. Dermatologic manifestations of Wegener granulomatosis, Inc.; c2011 [updated 2013 Oct 23; cited 2014 Jan 29]. Available from: http://emedicine.medscape.com/article/1085290.
- Erickson VR, Hwang PH: Wegener's granulomatosis: current trends in diagnosis and management. Curr Opin Otolaryngol Head Neck Surg 2007; 15:170–176.
- Fauci AS, Haynes BF, Katz P, Wolff SM. Wegener's granulomatosis: prospective clinical and therapeutic experience with 85 patients for 21 years. Ann Intern Med 1983; 98: 76–85.
- Faurschou M, Helleberg M, Obel N, Baslund B. Incidence of granulomatosis with polyangiitis (Wegener's) in Greenland and the Faroe Islands: epidemiology of an ANCA-associated vasculitic syndrome in two ethnically distinct populations in the North Atlantic area. Clin Exp Rheumatol 2013; 31 (1 Suppl 75): S52–55.
- Fernandes NC, Castilho M, Paes C, Macieira J. Granulomatose de Wegener localizada com manifestação ocular: relato de caso. An Bras Dermatol. 1998;73:107-10.
- Finkielman JD, Lee AS, Hummel AM et al. ANCA are detectible in nearly all patients with active severe Wegener's granulomatosis. Am. J. Med. 2007; 120: 643.e9–e14.
- Frascà GM, Zoumparidis NG, Borgnino LC, Neri L, Neri L, Vangelista A, Bonomini V. Combined treatment in Wegener's granulomatosis with crescentic glomerulonephritis – clinical course and long-term outcome. Int J Artif Organs, 1993, 16(1): 11–19.
- Georganas C, Ioakimidis D, Iatrou C, Vidalaki B, Iliadou K, Athanassiou P, Kontomerkos T. Relapsing Wegener's gra-nulomatosis:

successful treatment with cyclosporine-A. Clin Reumatol, 1996, 15(2):189–192.

- Gluth MB, Shinners PA, Kasperbauer JL. Subglottic stenosis associated with Wegener's granulomatosis. Laryngoscope 2003; 113(8):1304–7.
- Gottschlich S, Ambrosch P, Kramkowski D, Laudien M, Buchelt T, Gross WL, Hellmich B. Head and neck manifesta-tions of Wegener's granulomatosis. Rhinology, 2006, 44(4): 227–233.
- Hamada K, Nagai S, Kitaichi M, Jin G, Shigematsu M, Nagao T, Sato A, Mishima M. Cyclophosphamide-induced late-onset lung disease. Intern Med, 2003, 42(1):82–87.
- Haris M, Koulaouzidis A, Yasir M, Clark S, Kaleem M, Mallya R. Wegener's granulomatosis. CMAJ, 2008, 178(1):25–26.
- Hernández-Rodríguez J, Hoffman G.S, Koening CL. Surgical interventions and local therapy for Wegener's granulomatosis. Curr Opin Rheumatol 2010; 22: 29–36. doi: 10.1097/ BOR.0b013e328333e9e9.
- Hervier B, Pagnoux C, Renaudin K, Masseau A, Pottier P, Planchon B et al. Endobronchial stenosis in Wegener's granulomatosis. La Revue de médecine interne/fondée 2006; 27(6):453–7.
- Hilhorst M, Wilde B, van Paassen P, Winkens B, van Breda Vriesman P, Cohen Tervaert JW; Limburg Renal Registry. Improved outcome in anti-neutrophil cytoplasmic antibody (ANCA)-associated glomerulonephritis: a 30-year follow-up study. Nephrol Dial Transplant, 2013, 28(2):373–379.
- Hoffman GS, Thomas-Golbanov CK, Chan J, Akst LM, Eliachar I. Treatment of subglottic stenosis, due to Wegener's granulomatosis, with intralesional corticosteroids and dilation. J Rheumatol 2003; 30(5):1017–21.

- Holle JU, Laudien M, Gross WL. Clinical manifestations and treatment of Wegener's granulomatosis. Rheum. Dis Clin North Am 2010; 36: 507–526. doi: 10.1016/j.rdc.2010.05.008.
- Holle JU, Gross WL, Latza U, Nölle B, Ambrosch P, Heller M, Fertmann R, Reinhold-Keller E. Improved outcome in 445 patients with Wegener's granulomatosis in a German vasculitis center over four decades. Arthritis Rheum, 2011, 63(1):257–266.
- Jennette JC, Falk RJ, Bacon PA, Basu N, Cid MC, Ferrario F, et al. 2012 Revised International Chapel Hill Consensus Conference Nomenclature of Vasculitides. Arthritis Rheum. 2013;65:1-11.
- Jennings CR, Jones NS, Dugar J, Powell RJ, Lowe J. Wegener's granulomatosis – a review of diagnosis and treatment in 53 subjects. Rhinology, 1998, 36(4):188–191.
- Kallenberg CGM: Antineutrophil cytoplasmic antibodies (ANCA) and vasculitis. Clin Rheumatol 1990; 9(Suppl 1):132–135.
- Langford CA, Sneller MC, Hallahan CW, Hoffman GS, Kammerer WA, Talar-Williams C et al. Clinical features and therapeutic management of subglottic stenosis in patients with Wegener's granulomatosis. Arthritis Rheum 1996; 39(10):1754–60.
- Leavitt, RY, Fauci, AS, Bloch, DA et al. The American College of Rheumatology 1990 criteria for the classification of Wegener's granulomatosis. Arthritis Rheum , 1990; 33:1101–1102.
- Leavitt RY, Fauci AS. Less common manifestations and presentations of Wegener's granulomatosis. Curr Opin Rheumatol, 1992, 4(1):16–22.
- Lebovics RS, Hoffman GS, Leavitt RY, Kerr GS, Travis WD, Kammerer W et al. The management of subglottic stenosis in patients with Wegener's granulomatosis. Laryngoscope 1992; 102(12 Pt 1):1341–5.
- Lee AS, Finkielman JD, Peikert T, Hummel AM, Viss MA, Jacob GL et al. Agreement of anti-neutrophil cytoplasmic antibody measurements

obtained from serum and plasma. Clin Exp Immunol 2006; 146(1):15–20.

- Lutalo PM, D'Cruz DP. Diagnosis and classifcation of granulomatosis with polyangiitis (aka Wegener's granulomatosis). J Autoimmun. 2014;48-49:94-8.
- McDonald TJ, DeRemee RA, Kern EB, Harrison EG Jr. Nasal manifestations of Wegener's granulomatosis. Laryngoscope, 1974, 84(12):2101–2112.
- McDonald TJ, DeRemee RA. Wegener's granulomatosis. Laryngoscope, 1983, 93(2):220–231.
- McDonald TJ. Granulomatous diseases of the nose. In: English GM (ed). Otolaryngology. Vol. 2, J.B. Lippincott Co., Philadelphia, 1990, 1–14.
- McDonald TJ: Wegener's granulomatosis of the nose. In McCaffrey TV, editor: Systemic Disease and the Nasal Airway (Rhinology and Sinusology), New York, Thieme, 1993.
- Mokoka MC, Ullah K, Curran DR, O'Connor TM. Rare causes of persistent wheeze that mimic poorly controlled asthma. BMJ Case Rep, 2013.
- Morgan MD, Day CJ, Piper KP et al. Patients with Wegener's granulomatosis demonstrate a relative deficiency and functional impairment of T-regulatory cells. Immunol 2010; 130: 64–73. doi: 10.1111/j.1365-2567.2009.03213.x.
- Murty GE. Wegener's granulomatosis: otorhinolaryngological manifestations. Clin Otolaryngol Allied Sci, 1990, 15(4):385–393.
- Parra-García GD, Callejas-Rubio JL, Ríos-Fernández R, Sainz-Quevedo M, Ortego-Centeno N. Manifestaciones otorrinola-ringológicas de las vasculitis sistémicas. Acta Otorrinolaringol Esp, 2012, 63(4):303–310.
- Pereira DB, Amaral JLA, Szajubok JCM, Lima SMAL, Chahade WH. Otorhinolaryngologic manifestations of auto-immune rheumatic diseases. Rev Bras Reumatol, 2006, 46(2):118–125.

- Pires APBA, Sousa NJA, Sousa RCA, et al. Wegener's granulomatosis presenting with bilateral facial nerve palsy. Acta ORL 2008;26(4): 209–259.
- Polychronopoulos VS, Prakash UB, Golbin JM, Edell ES, Specks U. Airway involvement in Wegener's granulomatosis. Rheum Dis Clin North Am 2007; 33(4):755–75, vi.
- Prince JS, Duhamel DR, Levin DL, Harrell JH, Friedman PJ. Nonneoplastic lesions of the tracheobronchial wall: radiologic fi ndings with bronchoscopic correlation. Radiographics 2002; 22 Spec No:S215–30.
- Rasmussen N. L24. Local treatments of subglottic and tracheal stenoses in granulomatosis with polyangiitis (Wegener's). Presse Med 2013; 42: 571–574. doi: 10.1016/j.lpm.2013.01.024.
- Reinhold-Keller E, Kekow J, Schnabel A, Schwarz-Eywill M, Schmitt WH, Gross WL. Effectiveness of cyclophosphamide pulse treatment in Wegener's granulomatosis. Adv Exp Med Biol, 1993, 336:483–486.
- Reinhold-Keller E, Kekow J, Schnabel A, Schmitt WH, Heller M, Beigel A, Duncker G, Gross WL. Influence of disease mani-festation and antineutrophil cytoplasmic antibody titer on the response to pulse cyclophosphamide therapy in patients with Wegener's granulomatosis. Arthritis Rheum, 1994, 37(6):919–924.
- Regan MJ, Hellmann DB, Stone JH: Treatment of Wegener's granulomatosis. Rheum Dis Clin North Am 2001; 27(4):863–886.
- Rezende CEB, Rodrigues REC, Yoshimura R, Uvo IP, Rapoport PB. Wegener's granulomatosis: a case report. Rev Bras Otorrinolaringol 2003;69:261–265.
- Rhee EP, Laliberte KA, Niles JL. Rituximab as maintenance therapy for anti-neutrophil cytoplasmic antibody-associated vasculitis. Clin J Am Soc Nephrol 2010; 5: 1394–1400. doi: 10.2215/CJN.08821209.

- Rossini BAA, Bogaz EA, Yonamine FK, Testa JRG, Penido NdeO. Refractory otitis media as the first manifestation of Wegener's granulomatosis. Braz J Otorhinolaryngol 2010; 76(4):541.
- Sanchez-Cano D, Callejas-Rubio JL, Ortego-Centeno N: Effect of rituximab on refractory Wegener granulomatosis with predominant granulomatous disease. J Clin Rheumatol 2008; 14(2):92–93.
- Scalcon MRR, Pereira IA, Rachid Filho A, Paiva ES. Manifestação otológica localizada em paciente com granulomatose deWegener. Rev Bras Reumatol 2008;48(4):253–255.
- Screaton NJ, Sivasothy P, Flower CD, Lockwood CM. Tracheal involvement in Wegener's granulomatosis: evaluation using spiral CT. Clin Radiol 1998; 53(11):809–15.
- Seo P, Stone JH: The antineutrophil cytoplasmic antibodyassociated vasculitides. Am J Med 2004; 117:39–50.
- Solans-Laqué R, Bosch-Gil JA, Canela M, Lorente J, Pallisa E, Vilardell-Tarrés M. Clinical features and therapeutic management of subglottic stenosis in patients with Wegener's granulomatosis. Lupus 2008; 17: 832−836. doi:10.1177/0961203308089693
- Specks U, Wheatley CL, McDonald TJ, et al: Anticytoplasmic autoantibodies in the diagnosis and follow-up of Wegener's granulomatosis. Mayo Clin Proc 1989; 64:28–36.
- Springer J, Nutter B, Langford CA, Hoffman GS, Villa-Forte A. Granulomatosis with polyangiitis (Wegener's): impact of maintenance therapy duration. Medicine (Baltimore), 2014, 93(2):82–90.
- Stassen PM, Tervaert JW, Stegeman CA: Induction of remission in active anti-neutrophil cytoplasmic antibody–associated vasculitis with mycophenolate mofetil in patients who cannot be treated with cyclophosphamide. Ann Rheum Dis 66:798–802, 2007.

- Stegmayr BG, Gothefors L, Malmer B, Müller Wiefel DE, Nilsson K, Sundelin B. Wegener granulomatosis in children and young adults. A case study of ten patients. Pediatr Nephrol, 2000, 14(3):208–213.
- Strange C, Halstead L, Baumann M, Sahn SA. Subglottic stenosis in Wegener's granulomatosis: development during cyclophosphamide treatment with response to carbon dioxide laser therapy. Thorax 1990; 45(4):300–1.
- Summers RM, Aggarwal NR, Sneller MC, Cowan MJ, Wood BJ, Langford CA, Shelhamer JH. CT virtual bronchoscopy of the central airways in patients with Wegener's granulomatosis. Chest 2002;121(1):242-50.
- Taborda P, Taborda V. Granulomatose de Wegener. An Bras Dermatol. 1998;73:135-41.
- Takagi D, Nakamaru Y, Maguchi S, Furuta Y, Fukuda S. Otologic manifestations of Wegener's granulomatosis. Laryn-goscope, 2002, 112(9):1684–1690.
- Tami TA: Granulomatous diseases and chronic rhinosinusitis. Otolaryngol Clin North Am 2005; 38:1267–1278.
- Tomasson G, Davis JC, Hoffman GS, McCune WJ, Specks U, Spiera R, St Clair EW, Stone JH, Merkel PA. Brief report: The value of a patient global assessment of disease activity in granulomatosis with polyangiitis (Wegener's). Arthritis Rheu-matol, 2014, 66(2):428–432.
- Vartiainen E, Nuutinen J. Head and neck manifestations of Wegener's granulomatosis. Ear Nose Throat J, 1992, 71(9): 423–424; 427–428.
- Wegener F: Uber eine eigenartige Rhinogene granulomatose mit besonderer Beteiligung des Arteriensystems und der Nieren. Beitre Pathol Anat 1939; 102:36–68.
- Wolter NE, Ooi EH, Witterick IJ. Intralesional corticosteroid injection and dilatation provides effective management of subglottic stenosis in

Wegener's granulomatosis. Laryngoscope 2010; 120: 2452–2455. doi: 10.1002/lary.21121.
- Wung PK, Stone JH: Therapeutics of Wegener's granulomatosis. Nat Clin Pract Rheumatol 2006; 2:192–200.
- Zycinska K, Wardyn KA, Zielonka TM, Krupa R, Lukas W. Co-trimoxazole and prevention of relapses of PR3-ANCA positive vasculitis with pulmonary involvement. Eur J Med Res 2009; 14 (Suppl 4): 265–267.

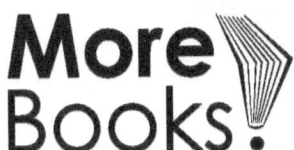
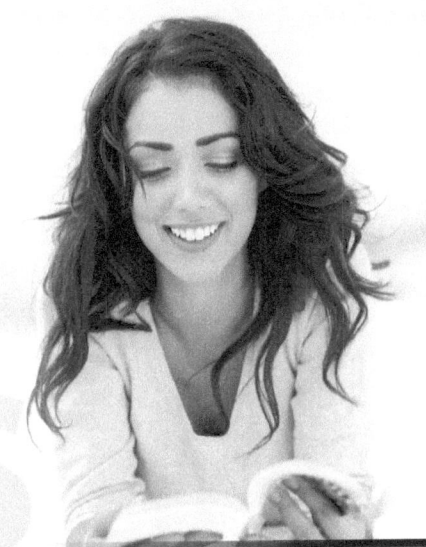

I want morebooks!

Buy your books fast and straightforward online - at one of the world's fastest growing online book stores! Environmentally sound due to Print-on-Demand technologies.

Buy your books online at
www.get-morebooks.com

Kaufen Sie Ihre Bücher schnell und unkompliziert online – auf einer der am schnellsten wachsenden Buchhandelsplattformen weltweit! Dank Print-On-Demand umwelt- und ressourcenschonend produziert.

Bücher schneller online kaufen
www.morebooks.de

OmniScriptum Marketing DEU GmbH
Heinrich-Böcking-Str. 6-8
D - 66121 Saarbrücken
Telefax: +49 681 93 81 567-9

info@omniscriptum.com
www.omniscriptum.com

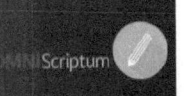